DIVINE HEALTH AFFIRMATIONS AGAINST MISCARRIAGE

.....A THERAPY THAT WORKS....

BY
IHEKE WILLIAMS

Unless otherwise indicated, all scripture quotations are taken from the King James Version of the Bible A key for other Bible versions used

NKJV	New King James Version
AMP	The Amplified Bible
TANT	The New Amplified Bible
TLB -	The Living Bible
CEV -	Contemporary English Version
NASB	New American Standard Version
GW -	God's Word version
ESV -	English Standard Version
NET -	New English Translation
ISV -	International Standard Version
NIV -	New International Version
MSG -	The Message Translation

<u>DEDICATION</u>

This Book is dedicated to Almighty God and to every married couple in the world.

TABLE OF CONTENT

WHAT IS MISCARRIAGE?

A **miscarriage** is the natural death of an embryo or fetus in the womb, before it is old enough to live on its own, outside the mother.

The medical words for a miscarriage are **spontaneous abortion.** ("Spontaneous" means something that a person did not expect to happen. An "abortion" is when a pregnancy ends early, before birth).

Among women who know they are pregnant, about 15-20% have miscarriages. (This means that up to 1 in every 5 women who know they are pregnant miscarries.) It is the most common complication (serious problem) that happens in early pregnancy in humans.

Source: Wikipedia

WHAT IS GOD'S SOLUTION

"...By His wounds ye have been healed.."
1 Peter 2:24

JESUS has already healed you over 2000 years ago.

You have NO business with Miscarriages.

You are Active and Fruitful because of all Jesus suffered on the cross for your sake.

For the next 31 days and forever, you will affirm this Blessing.

INSTRUCTIONS

That if thou shalt confess with thy mouth the Lord Jesus, and shalt believe in thine heart that God hath raised him from the dead, thou shalt be saved. – Romans 10:9

There has to be a connection with what you say and what you have in your heart.

For the affirmations to be effective, you will have to meditate on the scripture (1Peter 2:24) for 5 minutes, in your heart, and then affirm it with your mouth.

DAY 1
AFFIRMATION

Meditate on 1 Peter 2:24B for 5 minutes

"..By His stripes ye have been healed"

Now place your hands on your stomach and say the following words to yourself

"I HAVE BEEN HEALED THEREFORE, I AFFIRM THAT MY WOMB IS ACTIVE STRONG AND FRUITFUL!"

DAY 2
AFFIRMATION

Meditate on 1 Peter 2:24B
in your heart for 5 minutes

**"..By His stripes ye have
been healed"**

Now place your hands on your
stomach and say the following
words to yourself

**"I HAVE BEEN
HEALED THEREFORE,
I AFFIRM THAT MY
WOMB IS ACTIVE
AND FERTILE!"**

DAY 3
AFFIRMATION

Meditate on 1 Peter 2:24B in
your heart for 5 minutes

"..By His stripes ye have been
healed.."

Now place your hands on your
stomach and say the following words
to yourself

"I HAVE BEEN
HEALED THEREFORE,
I AFFIRM THAT MY
REPRODUCTIVE
ORGANS ARE ACTIVE
AND FRUITFUL!"

DAY 4
AFFIRMATION

Meditate on 1 Peter 2:24B in your heart for 5 minutes

"..By His stripes ye have been healed.."

Now place your hands on your stomach and say the following words to yourself

"I HAVE BEEN HEALED THEREFORE, I AFFIRM THAT MY OVULATION IS ACTIVE AND FRUITFUL!"

DAY 5
AFFIRMATION

Meditate on 1 Peter 2:24B in your heart for 5 minutes

"..By His stripes ye have been healed.."

Now place your hands on your stomach and say the following words to yourself

"I HAVE BEEN HEALED THEREFORE, I AFFIRM THAT MY OVARIES ARE ACTIVE AND FRUITFUL!"

DAY 6
AFFIRMATION

Meditate on 1 Peter 2:24B in your heart for 5 minutes

"..By His stripes ye have been healed"

Now place your hands on your stomach and say the following words to yourself

"I HAVE BEEN HEALED THEREFORE, I AFFIRM THAT MY HORMONES ARE ACTIVE, NORMAL, BALANCED AND FRUITFUL!"

DAY 7
AFFIRMATION

Meditate on 1 Peter 2:24B
in your heart for 5 minutes

" ..By His stripes ye have
been healed.."

Now place your hands on your
stomach and say the following
words to yourself

**"I HAVE BEEN
HEALED
THEREFORE, I
AFFIRM THAT MY
EGGS ARE ACTIVE,
FERTILE AND
FRUITFUL!"**

DAY 8
AFFIRMATION

Meditate on 1 Peter 2:24B
in your heart for 5 minutes

"..By His stripes ye have
been healed"

Now place your hands on your
stomach and say the following
words to yourself

**"I HAVE BEEN
HEALED
THEREFORE, I
AFFIRM THAT MY
FALLOPIAN TUBE IS
ACTIVE AND
FRUITFUL!"**

DAY 9
AFFIRMATION

Meditate on 1 Peter 2:24B in your heart for 5 minutes

"..By His stripes ye have been healed.."

Now place your hands on your stomach and say the following words to yourself

"I HAVE BEEN HEALED THEREFORE, I AFFIRM THAT I HAVE NO SEXUALLY TRANSMITTED INFECTIONS INSIDE MY BODY!"

DAY 10
AFFIRMATION

Meditate on 1 Peter 2:24B
in your heart for 5 minutes

"..By His stripes ye have
been healed"

Now place your hands on your
stomach and say the following
words to yourself

"I HAVE BEEN HEALED THEREFORE, I AFFIRM THAT I AM ACTIVE, STRONG AND FRUITFUL!"

DAY 11
AFFIRMATION

Meditate on 1 Peter 2:24B in your heart for 5 minutes

"..By His stripes ye have been healed"

Now place your hands on your stomach and say the following words to yourself

"I HAVE BEEN HEALED THEREFORE, I AFFIRM THAT MY IMMUNE SYSTEM IS ACTIVE AND STRONG!"

AFFIRMATION

Meditate on 1 Peter 2:24B in your heart for 5 minutes

"..By His stripes ye have been healed.."

Now place your hands on your stomach and say the following words to yourself

"I HAVE BEEN HEALED THEREFORE, I AFFIRM THAT MY UTERINE CONDITION IS PERFECT AND NORMAL!"

DAY 13
AFFIRMATION

Meditate on 1 Peter 2:24B
in your heart for 5 minutes

"..By His stripes ye have
been healed.."

Now place your hands on your
stomach and say the following
words to yourself

"I HAVE BEEN
HEALED
THEREFORE, I
AFFIRM THAT I DO
NOT HAVE
GENETIC
PROBLEMS!"

DAY 14
AFFIRMATION

Meditate on 1 Peter 2:24B in your heart for 5 minutes

"..By His stripes ye have been healed"

Now place your hands on your stomach and say the following words to yourself

"I HAVE BEEN HEALED THEREFORE, I AFFIRM THAT I DO NOT HAVE PELVIC DISEASE!"

DAY 15
AFFIRMATION

Meditate on 1 Peter 2:24B in
your heart for 5 minutes

"..By His stripes ye have
been healed"

Now place your hands on your
stomach and say the following
words to yourself

"I HAVE BEEN
HEALED THEREFORE,
I AFFIRM THAT MY
BODY IS STRONG
AND ACTIVE!"

DAY 16
AFFIRMATION

Meditate on 1 Peter 2:24B
in your heart for 5 minutes

"..By His stripes ye have
been healed"

Now place your hands on your
stomach and say the following
words to yourself

"I AFFIRM THAT MY BABY IS ACTIVE AND STRONG!"

DAY 17
AFFIRMATION

Meditate on 1 Peter 2:24B in your heart for 5 minutes

"..By His stripes ye have been healed"

Now place your hands on your stomach and say the following words to yourself

"I AFFIRM THAT MY REPRODUCTIVE ORGANS ARE ACTIVE AND FRUITFUL!"

DAY 18
AFFIRMATION

Meditate on 1 Peter 2:24B
in your heart for 5 minutes

**"..By His stripes ye have
been healed"**

Now place your hands on your
stomach and say the following
words to yourself

"I AFFIRM THAT MY BABY IS ACTIVE AND FRUITFUL!"

DAY 19
AFFIRMATION

Meditate on 1 Peter 2:24B
in your heart for 5 minutes

**"..By His stripes ye have
been healed"**

Now place your hands on your
stomach and say the following
words to yourself

**" I AFFIRM THAT
MY BABY IS
HEALTHY AND
STRONG!"**

DAY 20
AFFIRMATION

Meditate on 1 Peter 2:24B
in your heart for 5 minutes

**"..By His stripes ye have
been healed"**

Now place your hands on your
stomach and say the following
words to yourself

"I AFFIRM THAT MY BODY IS ACTIVE AND FRUITFUL!"

DAY 21
AFFIRMATION

Meditate on 1 Peter 2:24B in your heart for 5 minutes

"..By His stripes ye have been healed"

Now place your hands on your stomach and say the following words to yourself

"I AFFIRM THAT I AM ACTIVE AND STRONG FOREVER!"

DAY 22
AFFIRMATION

Meditate on 1 Peter 2:24B in your heart for 5 minutes

"..By His stripes ye have been healed"

Now place your hands on your stomach and say the following words to yourself

"I AFFIRM THAT MY BABY IS HEALTHY AND STRONG!"

DAY 23
AFFIRMATION

Meditate on 1 Peter 2:24B
in your heart for 5
minutes

**"..By His stripes ye have
been healed"**

Now place your hands on your
stomach and say the following
words to yourself

**"I AFFIRM THAT
MY BABY DOES
NOT HAVE ANY
MEDICAL
CONDITION!"**

DAY 24
AFFIRMATION

Meditate on 1 Peter 2:24B in your heart for 5 minutes

"..By His stripes ye have been healed"

Now place your hands on your stomach and say the following words to yourself

"I AFFIRM THAT MY REPRODUCTIVE ORGANS ARE ACTIVE AND FRUITFUL!"

DAY 25
AFFIRMATION

Meditate on 1 Peter 2:24B
in your heart for 5 minutes

**"..By His stripes ye have
been healed"**

Now place your hands on your
stomach and say the following
words to yourself

"I AFFIRM THAT
MY BABY IS ACTIVE
AND STRONG!"

DAY 26
AFFIRMATION

Meditate on 1 Peter 2:24B
in your heart for 5 minutes

**"..By His stripes ye have
been healed"**

Now place your hands on your
stomach and say the following
words to yourself

"I AFFIRM THAT MY
BODY IS STRONG
AND ACTIVE
FOREVER!"

DAY 27
AFFIRMATION

Meditate on 1 Peter 2:24B in your heart for 5 minutes

"..By His stripes ye have been healed"

Now place your hands on your stomach and say the following words to yourself

"I AFFIRM THAT MY BABY IS STRONG AND ACTIVE!"

DAY 28
AFFIRMATION

Meditate on 1 Peter 2:24B
in your heart for 5 minutes

"..By His stripes ye have
been healed"

Now place your hands on your
stomach and say the following
words to yourself

"I AFFIRM THAT
MY BODY IS
ACTIVE AND
STRONG!"

DAY 29
AFFIRMATION

Meditate on 1 Peter 2:24B in your heart for 5 minutes

"..By His stripes ye have been healed"

Now place your hands on your stomach and say the following words to yourself

"I AFFIRM THAT MY BABY IS ACTIVE AND STRONG!"

DAY 30
AFFIRMATION

Meditate on 1 Peter 2:24B
in your heart for 5 minutes

**"..By His stripes ye have
been healed"**

Now place your hands on your
stomach and say the following
words to yourself

**"I AFFIRM THAT MY
BODY IS NORMAL,
ACTIVE AND
FRUITFUL!"**

DAY 31
AFFIRMATION

Meditate on 1 Peter 2:24B
in your heart for 5 minutes

"..By His stripes ye have
been healed"

Now place your hands on your
stomach and say the following
words to yourself

"I AFFIRM THAT
MY BABY IS
NORMAL, ACTIVE
AND STRONG
FOREVER!"

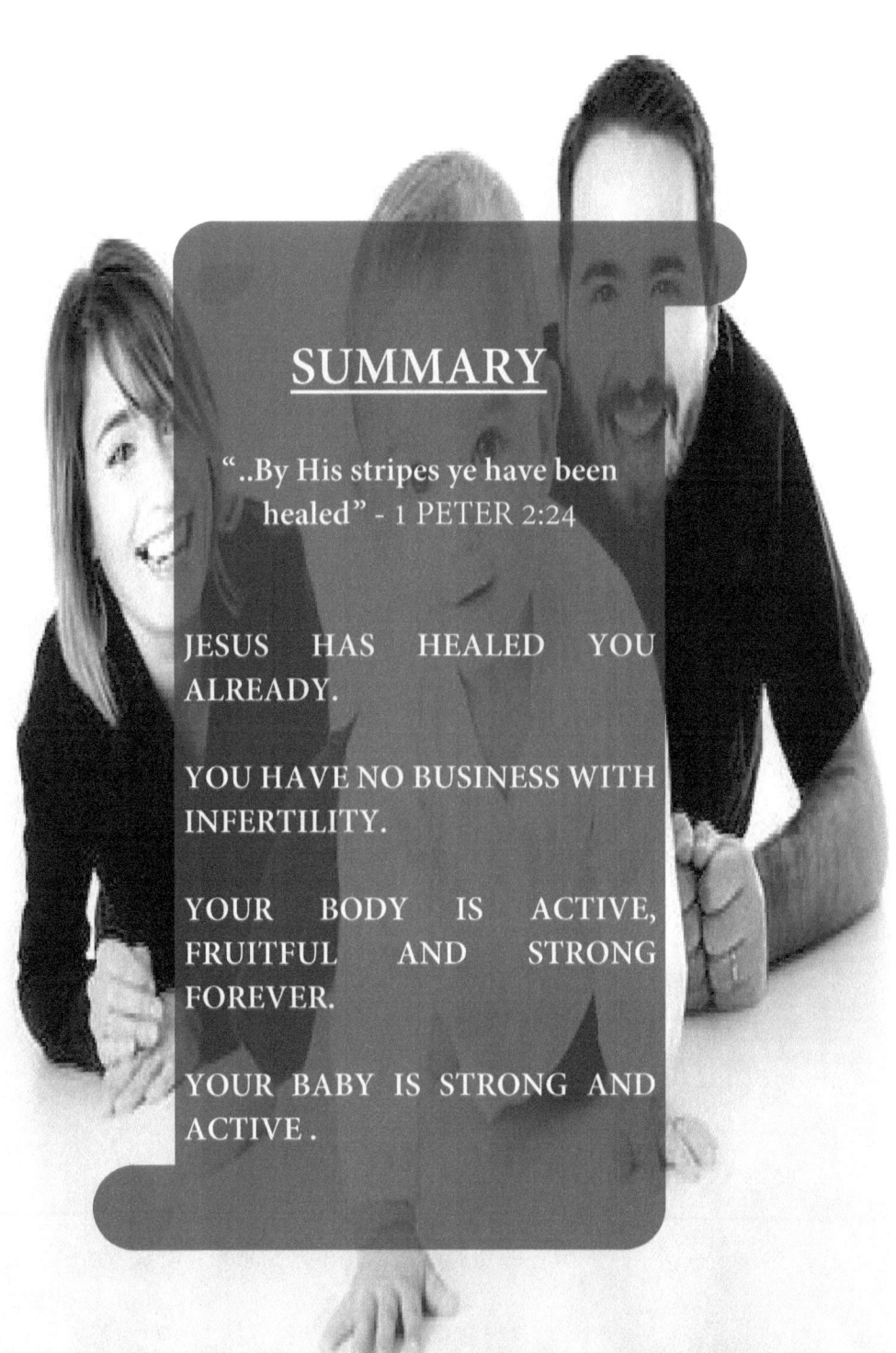

SUMMARY

"..By His stripes ye have been healed" - 1 PETER 2:24

JESUS HAS HEALED YOU ALREADY.

YOU HAVE NO BUSINESS WITH INFERTILITY.

YOUR BODY IS ACTIVE, FRUITFUL AND STRONG FOREVER.

YOUR BABY IS STRONG AND ACTIVE .

PRAYER FOR SALVATION

We believe that you have been blessed and that you want to receive eternal life that God has made available to everyone who believes in his love and his grace which He expressed lavishly through His Son Jesus Christ.

"For God so loved the world, that He gave his only begotten Son, that whosoever believeth in him should not perish, but have everlasting life." - John 3:16

Say this prayer to God and believe it with your heart

"Father, I believe that you gave me your only Son to die for my sin. I believe you raised Him from the dead. I declare that your son, Jesus Christ is the Lord of my life. I receive eternal life and I receive the Holy Spirit. I am saved forever.in Jesus name. I am so Happy that today and forever, I am your child. Amen ".

Congratulations, you are now a child of God Halleluyah!! — John 1:12

OTHER INFORMATION

Please share your testimonies via the following handles;

ihekewilliams@gmail.com
+2348061530541

Other Books written by the author includes
Dad, Pray for your Daughter
Mum, Pray for your Daughter
Mum, pray for your Son
Don't stop the flow of the Blessing
Daddy's Prayers
Mummy's Prayers
Divine Health Affirmation Against Cancer
Divine Health Affirmation Against Asthma
Divine Health Affirmation Series

ABOUT THE AUTHOR

Iheke Williams is a firm follower and disciple of the Lord Jesus Christ. He is a passionate minister of the grace of our Lord and savior Jesus Christ and has brought the reality of the divine life of Christ into the lives of so many.

Iheke Williams has a calling to communicate the gospel of Christ with simplicity and to show the world how to activate the eternal life of God that is in us already which includes Divine health, Divine righteousness, Divine security and Divine prosperity.

As you read this book and other books written by Iheke Williams you will literally begin to function and manifest the life of God that is already inside you to the glory of God the Father who is the author of all grace and mercy. Amen

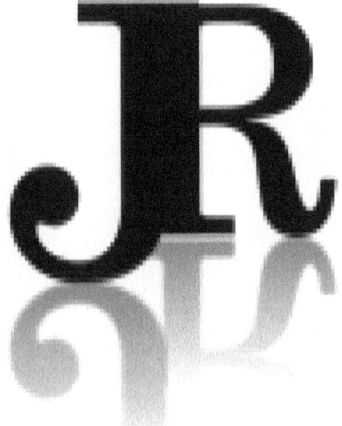